Uni

Caring for our loved ones
living with dementia

United

Caring for our loved ones
living with dementia

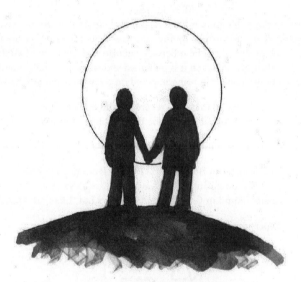

Gina Awad

Illustrated by Tony Husband

ROBINSON

ROBINSON

First published in Great Britain in 2022 by Robinson

3 5 7 9 8 6 4

A CIP catalogue record for this book is
available from the British Library

ISBN: 978-1-47214-651-9

Typeset in Bembo and Gotham Rounded by
SX Composing DTP, Rayleigh, Essex SS6 7EF
Printed and bound in Great Britain by Clays Ltd, Elcograf S.p.A.'

Papers used by Robinson are from well-managed forests
and other responsible sources

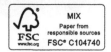

MIX
Paper from
responsible sources
FSC® C104740

Robinson
An imprint of
Little, Brown Book Group
Carmelite House
50 Victoria Embankment
London EC4Y 0DZ

An Hachette UK Company
www.hachette.co.uk

www.littlebrown.co.uk

Dedicated to my younger sister, Heidi, who had a ruptured brain aneurysm last year and is recovering well. At only eleven months apart, we're like twins; she's my best friend and I love her to the moon and back.

Contents

Contents

Foreword

I have learned a lot about dementia through my own experience of living with a family member with Alzheimer's over many years, and also through my involvement in raising several millions of pounds for research into this complex condition.

Society has been – and remains – far too inclined to dismiss dementia as an inevitable disease of old people, and so one that doesn't warrant the focus and attention given to other life-threatening conditions such as cancer. This could not be more wrong.

The reality is that dementia affects people of all ages and can have life-changing consequences that may last a decade or more.

Dementia doesn't just affect the individual but their family members and other people around them, and its impact on all of them can be devastating.

Sadly, one in three people alive today will be diagnosed with dementia, yet the funding for research is minuscule – while financial provision for the care of those affected is almost non-existent.

Funding long-term specialist care is a bottomless pit and, as a result, responsibility falls overwhelmingly on family members and friends acting as unpaid carers – and on care homes run on a shoestring.

Diagnosis of dementia is difficult: it may be many years before a diagnosis is reached, and many people go undiagnosed to the end.

It is important to recognise that the condition is not just about memory loss but can include difficulties with thinking, problem solving or language, as well as changes in personality and mood. As the true stories in this book show, these changes can be gradual and can have a huge impact on relationships if their cause is not understood.

I hope that this excellent book will help readers recognise and understand the early signs of dementia, and the changes that it brings about. Even after a diagnosis, which might explain initial behavioural changes, there are a whole series of further changes and stages that must be recognised and accepted.

For those living with and caring for loved ones with dementia, the most important thing is that impatience, irritation – and even despair – should be replaced with understanding, compassion and kindness.

Most educational resources shy away from describing the final stages of dementia, which can last for years, but it is important that they are also recognised, planned for and addressed by family members. You can find more information about the various stages of this illness by visiting https://www.alz.org/alzheimers-dementia/stages.

I am really grateful to Gina Awad and Tony Husband for researching, writing and illustrating the moving case studies of family carers featured in this book. I am sure they will help many people by raising awareness of dementia, and increasing understanding of how we all need to be prepared to recognise the symptoms and respond to them with empathy and love.

Sir Malcolm Walker CBE

Introduction

Over the years, I have witnessed family carers* struggle to meet the needs of their loved ones whilst neglecting their own. A myriad of overwhelming feelings can arise, including guilt for not being good enough and fear of getting it wrong, leading to immense frustration and loneliness.

However, they are doing the best they can with limited resources and often have no option but to educate themselves and attempt to navigate the intricate care system.

This has to change.

Dementia is not going away and it is one of the biggest health and social care challenges of this century. According to the World Alzheimer Report 2021, approximately fifty-six million people are living with dementia. These figures represent those formally diagnosed. What about those who are not?

This then raises the question of how many families are caring for their loved ones. We can only surmise.

Whilst the global search to find a cure gathers momentum, innovative practice continues to flourish and peer support increases, it still remains essential that as a society we seek to understand dementia and the impact it has on individuals and families. Engaging communities to work together for people living with dementia and their families is what drives my passion.

The idea of creating a book illustrating the range of varied experiences of families caring for their loved ones was born in the autumn of 2020.

This book was inspired by stories of isolation and loneliness during the global pandemic, alongside the new ways people found to connect with each other. It became vital to give families living with dementia a platform to share their personal stories and learning.

I have worked with Tony Husband, the wonderful cartoonist for this book, on several dementia-related projects over the past five years. Tony's illustrations tell the stories with such eloquence, heart and sensitivity that readers will come away smiling, moved and nodding with recognition.

Much of 2021 was spent in conversation with families on Zoom; listening, reflecting and working with Tony to create imagery that evoked the heart of their experiences. We acknowledged the responsibility, wishing to represent our contributors to the best of our ability. We knew that, told well, each individual story would be both unique and universal.

With the exception of John and Nobby, whose story is in the public domain due to Nobby's profile, we have made the difficult decision to anonymise names throughout as it would otherwise be impossible to guarantee the privacy and consent of everyone indirectly involved in each tale. However, each contributor has chosen their own pseudonym. Sienna's Story is the only tale not directly told by a real person; this is a composite story based on my own experiences and those of many professional carers who have shared with me over the years.

I hope these personal and heartfelt contributions provide an emotional and practical resource for everyone affected by dementia. Equally as important, Tony and I hope this book is part of the journey towards a society that responds to dementia with compassion and understanding.

Collaborating with these wonderfully caring, diverse families has been the most humbling of experiences. It has been evident throughout that they are partners in care, learning as they go along and striving to empower their loved ones to live as well as possible.

We thank you all from the bottom of our hearts for sharing so generously. We sincerely hope we have done your stories justice, with the utmost of sensitivity. We salute you for all you have done and will continue to do. Together we are United.

Many times, people with dementia and their families have expressed to me how they feel emotionally when we connect. I will sign off with this beautiful quote which offers so much truth to me and encapsulates perfectly how a felt sense of meaningful connection can last forever:

'People will forget what you said, people will forget what you did, but people will never forget how you made them feel' **Maya Angelou**

Gina Awad BEM

*Although the term 'carer' is used throughout the book, I acknowledge this word does not sit well with everyone and not everyone identifies as such. First and foremost, the relationship takes precedence. However, many people find that not identifying with the term can make accessing support very difficult.

Kate and Fred's Story

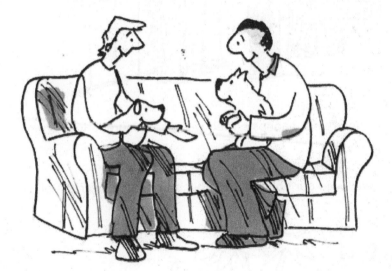

Kate's life changed when her husband Fred was diagnosed with dementia.

She had to adapt and learn new skills.

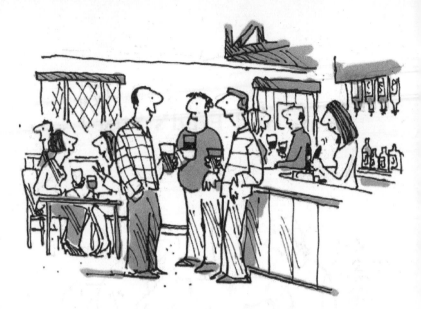

Before his diagnosis, Fred was a social, gregarious type.

We loved our holidays together. We went all over the place.

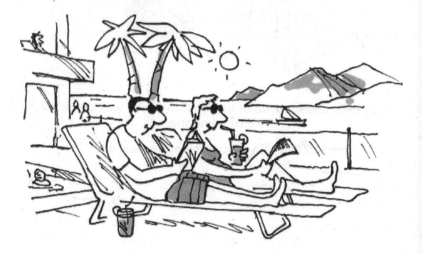

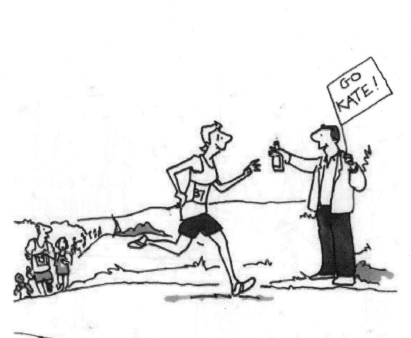

He supported me on my many marathons
with a cheer and a wave.

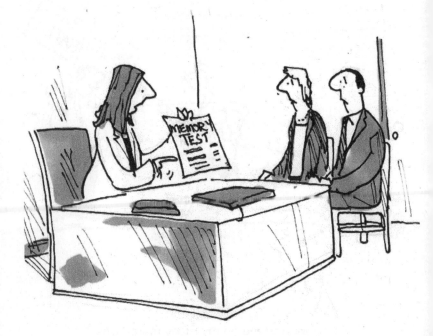

But with his diagnosis of vascular dementia,
things began to change for us.

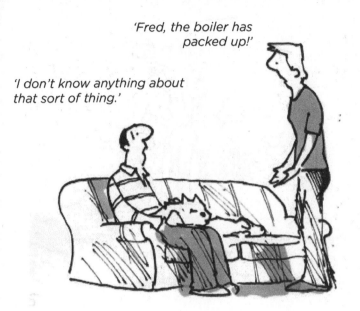

It was different for us then. The responsibilities were mine.
I had to learn quickly.

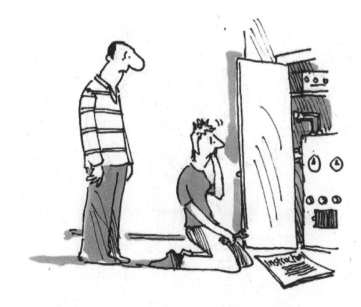

5

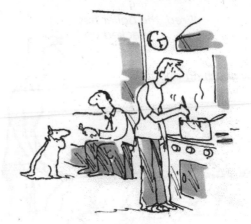

Fred used to love cooking; he was a great cook!
Sadly, I'm not, but I'm learning . . .

Some things can be difficult.

'Time for a shower, Fred.'

'I'm not going in there!'

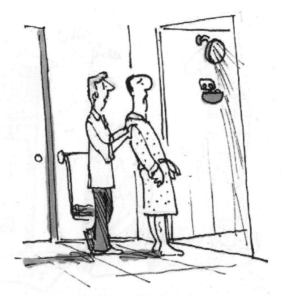

'Evening, Fred; your pint sir!'

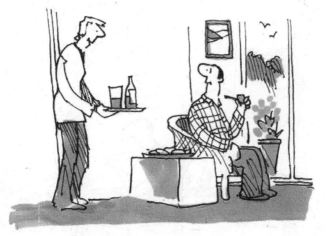

But by giving him a routine, like recreating his evening pint at the pub, he feels comfortable and content.

We have amazing carers who come on a rota system. They're fabulous. Fred's got to know them now and recognises their faces.

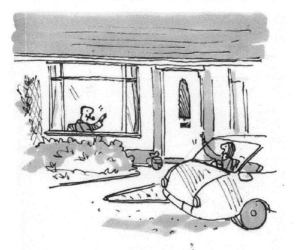

'Here we are, Fred, snack time!'

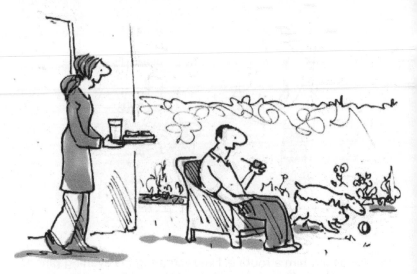

Fred and I think the world of them.

It was so important to me that I could find my own space and be independent, if only for a short time.

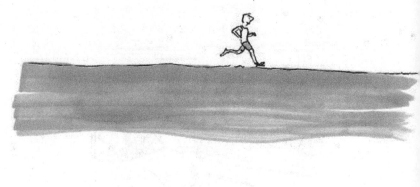

'Why have you only eaten half?'

'Because it's on the wrong side of the plate!'

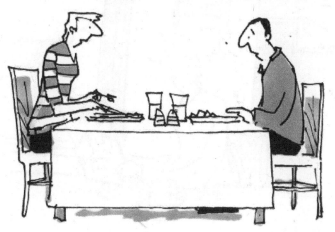

I noticed Fred would leave portions of his meals.

I realised he left the food on the side of the plate furthest from him. I served the next meal as a mix of quarter-sized portions. He ate three of the four. There's always something new to learn.

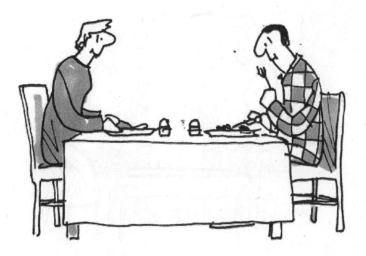

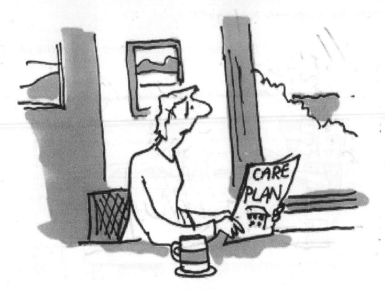

I sometimes feel angry and guilty. Dare I think of respite? Am I being selfish? Doubts are constant.

But through it all, we are together.
Not the us that was, but a different us.

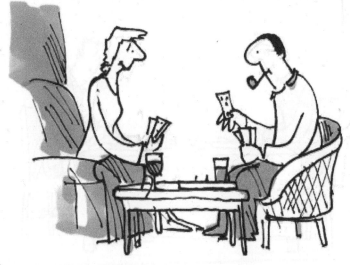

'Lunchtime, folks!'

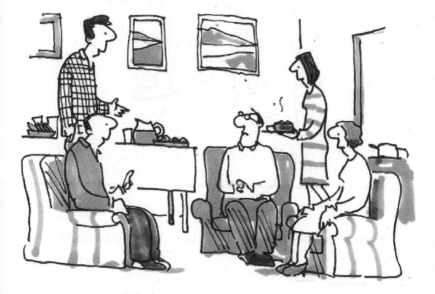

I discovered a wonderful initiative, so now once a week Fred is
collected by a host and taken to their home with up to three
people with dementia and similar interests. It's a break, and a
different experience. Fred really enjoys it
and there's a home-cooked meal too.

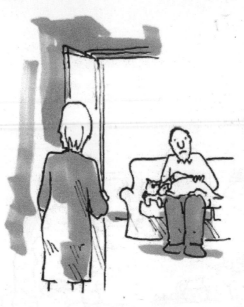

But those dark feelings of failure, ineptitude
and inadequacy often recur. I asked Fred once . . .

'Can you imagine anything worse than me as your carer?'

'Yes, you not being my carer.'

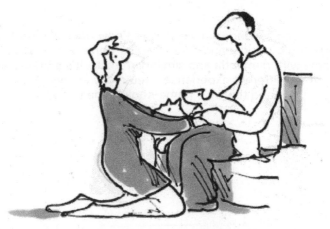

John and Nobby's Story

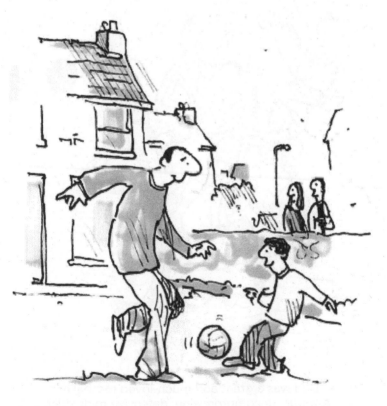

John and his family cared for their dad when he was diagnosed. They also began an important campaign to raise awareness of the dangers of heading a football.

'Great header, Nobby!'

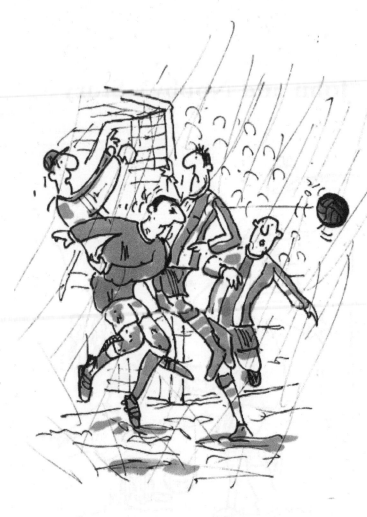

Dad was a great and much-loved footballer.
A tough, uncompromising, defensive midfielder.
He won a European Cup, a World Cup and much more.
He also won the heart of a nation.

'I'm sorry to tell you that you have dementia, Mr Stiles.'

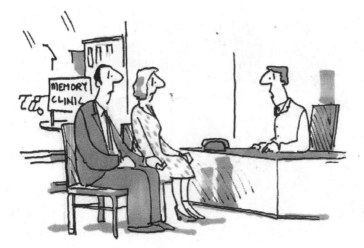

As a family, we decided to keep the news to ourselves
to protect Dad's profile. Life carried on regardless.

'Hello!'

'Grandad!!'

'Hi!'

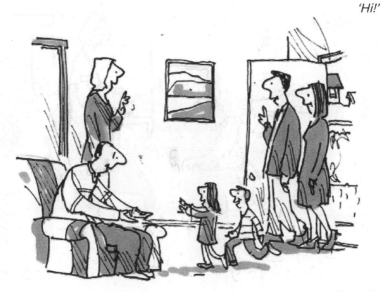

15

'So, Sir Matt walks in . . . '

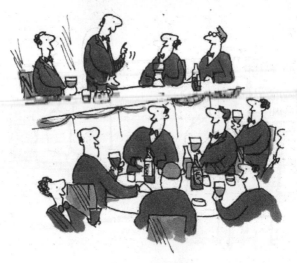

Dad had been a popular and in-demand public speaker
for many years.

But as the dementia progressed, Dad became more and more
confused. I was able to prompt him when his stories faltered.

'So Bobby, er, and er . . . '

'Georgie, Dad – Georgie Best!'

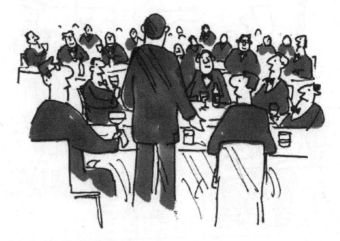

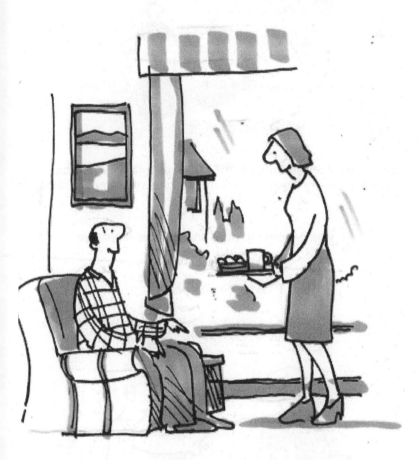

Sadly, things became too difficult, and Dad retired from the circuit.

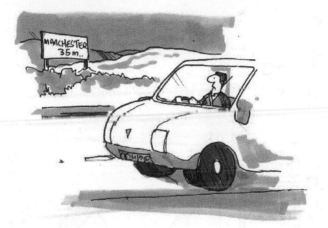

We were worried about Mum. Dad was totally reliant on her. My trips over to see them were fraught with concern about how things would be.

He was becoming more anxious, paranoid even. He was frightened.

'Where's she gone?'

'Mum's making us a cuppa, Dad. She'll be back soon, don't worry.'

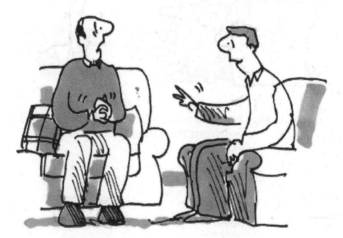

'*World Cup-winner Nobby Stiles has been diagnosed with dementia.*'

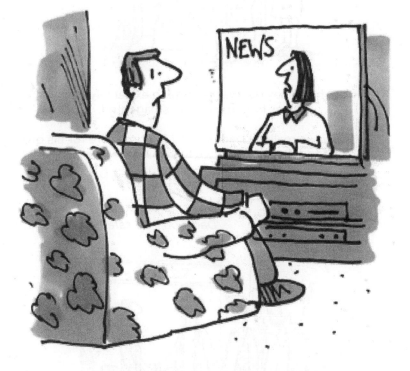

We decided as a family to go public with Dad's story. We didn't want people speculating.

'Where am I? What's going on? I need to go now!!!'

'It's OK, Dad, it's OK.'

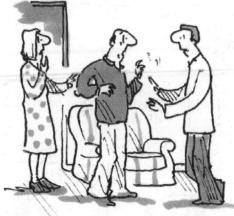

By now, his behaviour was becoming extremely worrying.
It was hard to see him so agitated.

Eventually, we realised Dad needed full-time care for his own
good. But the guilt we felt was unbearable.

'Where are we?'

'Dad, you'll be safe here, I promise.'

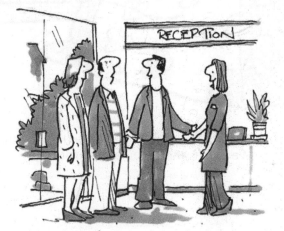

'Cup of tea, Nobby?'

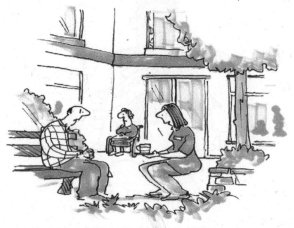

Dad remained agitated and restless, but was receiving
the specialised 24/7 treatment he needed.

Even as he deteriorated, he still loved our regular visits . . . and
so did we!

'Hi Dad, let's watch some football?'

'Sounds good!'

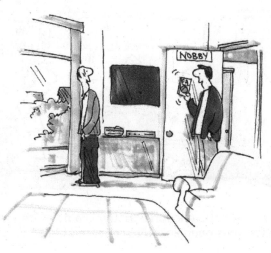

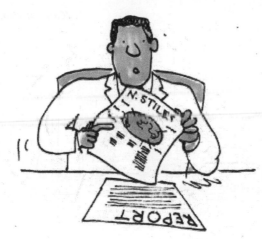

When Dad passed away, we decided as a family to donate his brain to medicine. The results that came back shocked and angered us. Years of heading a football had damaged and disturbed his brain. It turned out he had chronic traumatic encephalopathy (CTE).*

We felt it was our duty to raise awareness for Dad and other footballers who are literally putting their lives at risk heading a football.

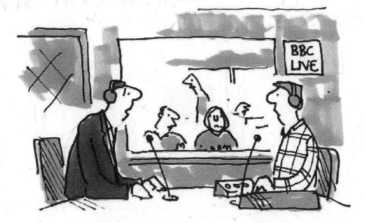

*Chronic traumatic encephalopathy is a neurodegenerative disease that has been linked to repeated blows to the head.

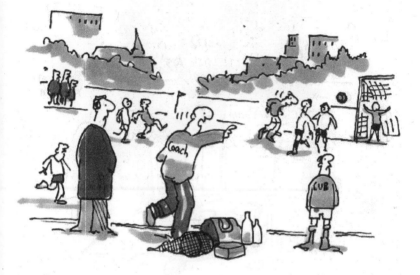

Sadly, heading is still an intrinsic part of football at all levels.

'Dad, is that my sandwich? You didn't want one! You said you weren't hungry!'

'Did I say that, son? Oh, sorry, I forgot.'

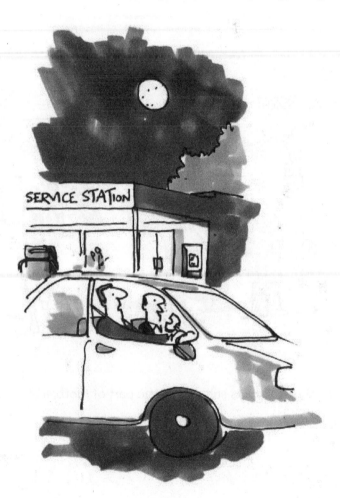

For me, travelling home from gigs listening to Dad's wonderful football stories – great tales from his remarkable career – was a joy, and created memories I will treasure for the rest of my life. My mate, my Dad, I miss you.

Penny and Emma's Story

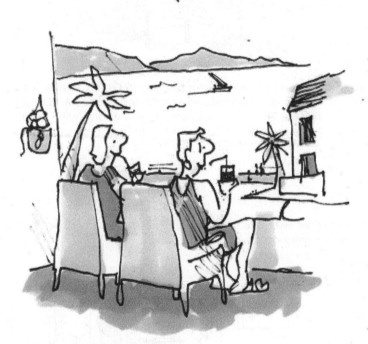

Penny and Emma lived contented lives in Gran Canaria, but a diagnosis of dementia meant rethinking their future.

'Go for a walk? Emma, you've asked me half a dozen times. Each time, I've said we'll go when I've finished this.'

'No, I haven't!'

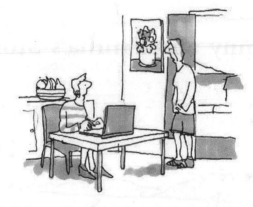

We'd been living and working happily in Gran Canaria for over twenty years. We had settled comfortably there and enjoyed the lifestyle. But there was something wrong with Emma. She kept repeating herself and her moods changed rapidly. It wasn't like her at all.

'Ready for that walk?'

'Walk? What walk? No, I don't want to go for a walk with you, thank you very much.'

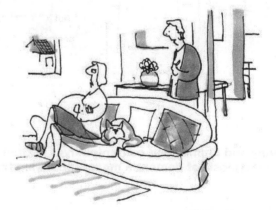

'What's wrong, Emma?'

'I don't know, but I want to go back to England.'

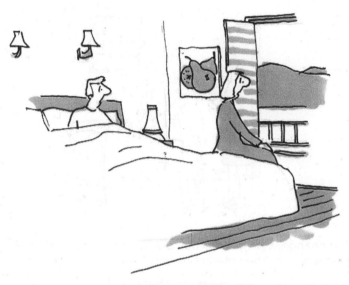

Emma became unsettled. She wanted to leave Gran Canaria even though we had a wonderful life there. We started looking for properties in England.

We came back to England for a fresh start, hoping the change would help Emma.

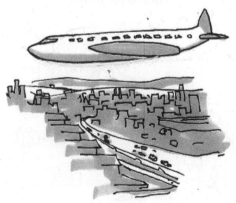

'Erm, Emma, the cutlery is in the kitchen drawer.'

'Oh yes, silly me.'

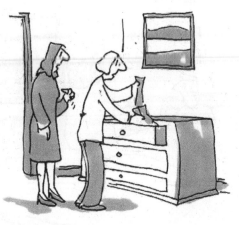

The change was hard for her. She didn't settle in at all at our new house. She couldn't remember where anything was. Her sister saw the confusion clearly.

The atmosphere in the house was often tense and uneasy. Things just flared up out of nowhere.

'What's wrong now? Where are you going?'

'I'm going for a walk!'

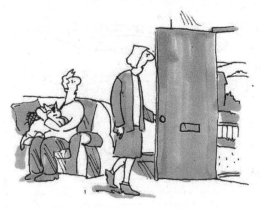

'This is a leaflet that explains dementia. We'll see you in a year.'

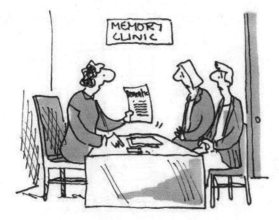

I realised I needed to seek professional advice and we eventually got a formal diagnosis. Emma had Alzheimer's, but the help we were offered was minimal.

We were on our own with little information, help or guidance. It was scary.

'Please don't put me in a care home, will you?'

'Of course I won't.'

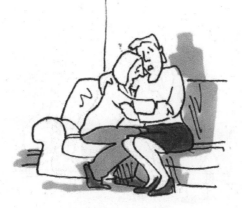

'If Emma has Alzheimer's, I strongly suggest you get power of attorney. This means you can act on her behalf if needed.'

'I hadn't even given it a thought, thank you.'

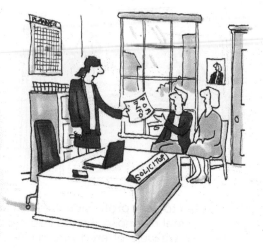

There was no guidance, so we sought advice from a solicitor.

We had to learn from friends and charities that Emma was entitled to attendance allowance. I knew from experience that, because of my savings, I wouldn't be granted carer's allowance.

'It's so unfair! I've worked and paid my taxes and saved all of my life!'

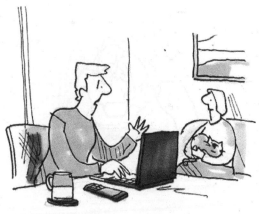

'We'd like to share with you what has helped us and made a difference.'

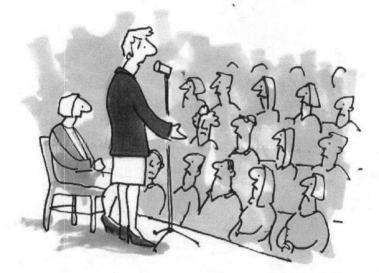

We got connected to a dementia charity and were asked to speak about our journey at a dementia conference. We felt a part of something. We weren't alone.

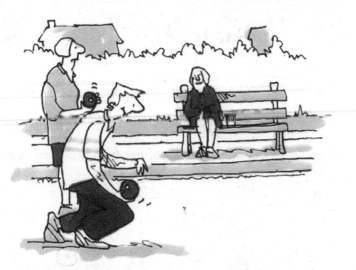

We had good times together and were still very close. I love my bowls and Emma would come along to watch and support me.

We would often go and visit the sheep in the fields near our home, which we both found very relaxing.

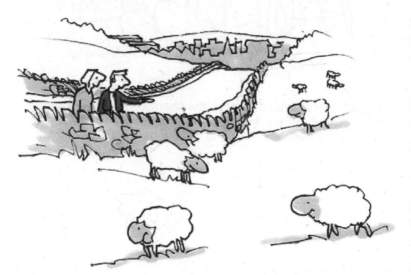

'Oh Alexa, where is Penny?'

'Penny has nipped to the shop. She will be back in ten minutes.'

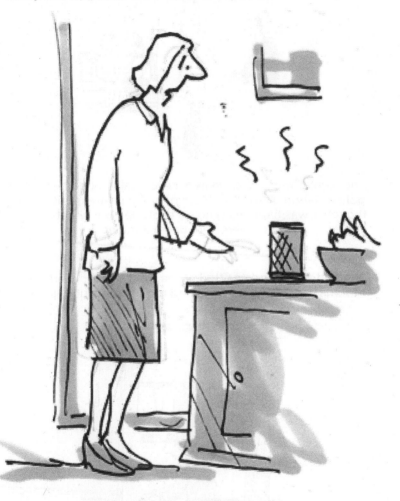

We had Alexa connected to reassure Emma if I was out
at any time.

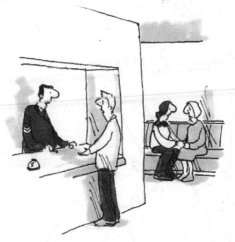

One night, Emma disappeared. I eventually found her at the police station. She'd told them of a bad past experience as though it was happening now. I explained our situation and they were very understanding.

We had a sensor pad fitted at the front door to alert me if Emma decided to go out. I had to take precautions now.

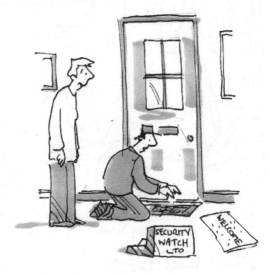

SECURITY
WATCH
LTD

WELCOME

'Oh look, can we go there soon?'

'I hope so. We should. Shouldn't we?'

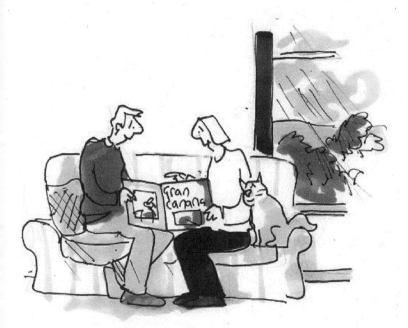

But we have decided we need to be back in Gran Canaria.
We miss it so much – the climate, our friends, everything,
actually . . .

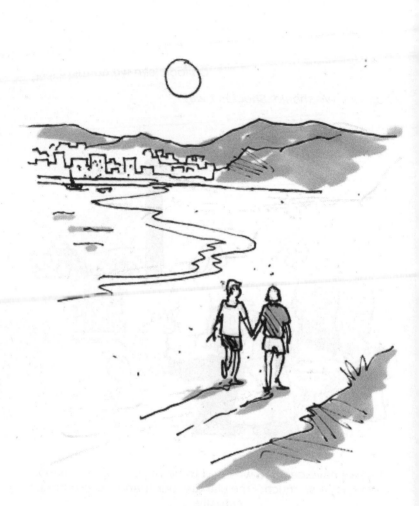

We will go back. We'll be together in the place we love,
the place where we are happiest.

Maya and Meera's Story

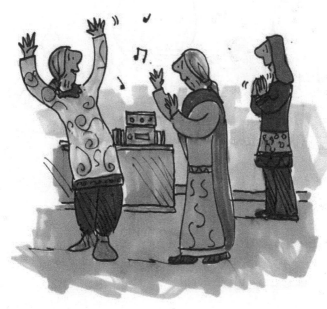

The physical distance was difficult between Maya and her mum, so Meera moved in with the family.

'*Where are we? Why are we here?*'

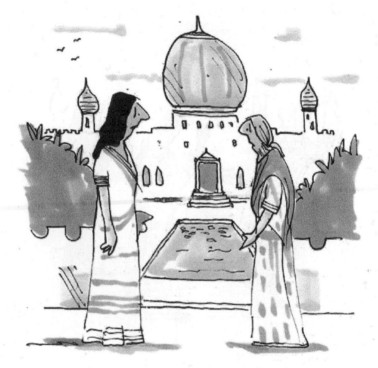

On a trip to India, my sister noticed a difference in Mum.
She was confused, disorientated and very forgetful.

'Mum, what are you doing? We've a table booked – we're taking you for dinner!'

'Oh, are you? I must have forgotten. I was just making dinner now.'

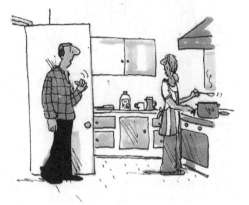

Back home in London, Mum lived on her own. My brothers visited often. They too noticed a big difference in her.

My brother was so concerned that he took her to the doctor, who immediately connected her with social services.

'Oh hi, it's Dr Harper here . . . '

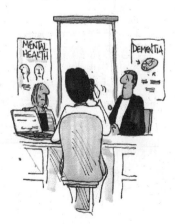

'Here we are, a nice cup of tea.'

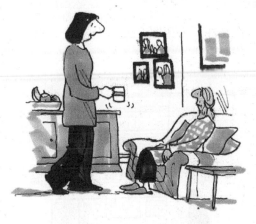

A lady came to sit with Mum, to chat and keep her company. My brothers had busy lives and found it hard to be there as much as they wanted to.

Mum had been diagnosed with dementia. She was obviously vulnerable. Something had to be done.

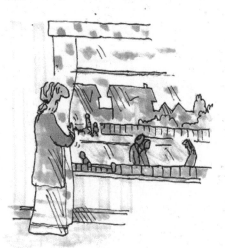

'Well, Mum, this is your room. Do you like it?'

'This isn't my room!'

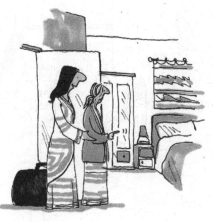

It was agreed between us that when she came north for a family occasion, instead of going back, she would stay with us.

It was a struggle at first, but we settled into a routine. My clever husband had researched all the benefits and allowances we were due. It wasn't easy gleaning information from the authorities.

'See, here's something else we weren't told about.'

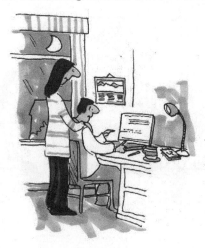

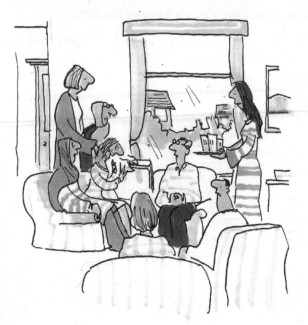

We'd been introduced to a fantastic local dementia group. Mum loved it. She was the life and soul, chatting away to anyone who'd listen.

She loved dancing and singing.

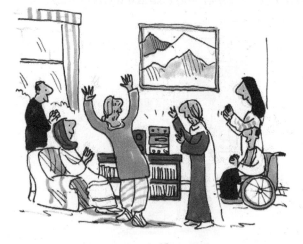

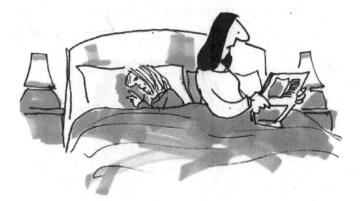

We had many challenges, though. She had hallucinations about people in her room. She was only comfortable and able to sleep when I slept with her.

She would hide things like money, pens, jewellery . . . I actually found her precious ring under the bed. I kept it safe, but she never asked for it.

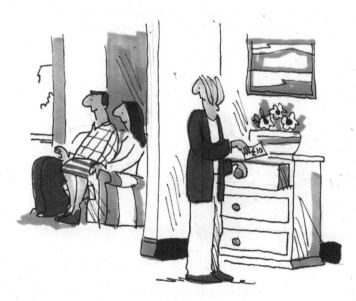

'I can't do this! How do you do this?!'

'Let's find something else for you to wear, Mum.'

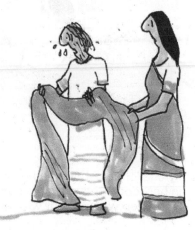

It became too difficult for Mum to put her sari on, and it was upsetting her. We decided casual clothes would be less stressful.

As the dementia advanced, she stopped speaking English. She forgot how to speak or understand it.

'તમે વિદેશી ભાષા કેમ બોલો છો?'*

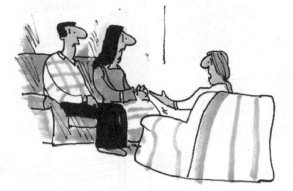

'Why are you speaking a foreign language?'

ઓહ મમ, આવો અને મારી સાથે બેસો.'*

મારે જવું છે, મને જવા દો!'**

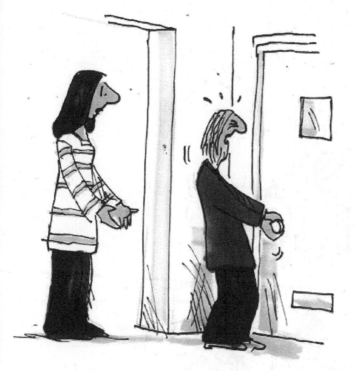

At times, she would stand at the door, banging on it and crying that she wanted to go home. It was heart-breaking and brought me to tears.

*'Oh Mum, come and sit down with me.'

**'I want to go . . . let me go!'

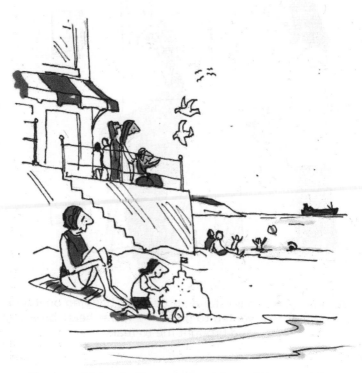

She loved trips to the countryside and the seaside.

આભાર, તે મારા માટે છે?'*

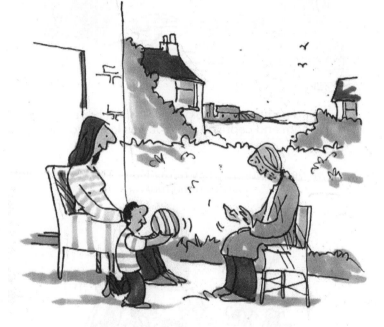

Visits from her great-grandson cheered her up. He made her smile, although we needed to make sure he didn't tire her out too much.

*'Thank you, is that for me?'

ते महान माता छे .'*

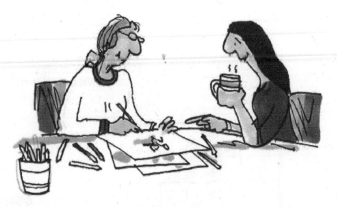

Mum loved painting and colouring. It gave her peace and freedom and captivated her. It was lovely to see.

I treasure her paintings. They're my Mum. They're her spirit. They're mine forever.

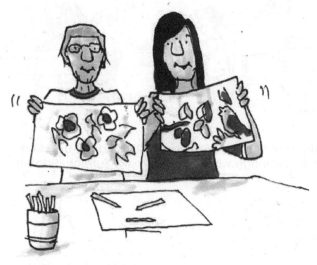

*'That's great, Mum.'

Cuthy and Roopwati's Story

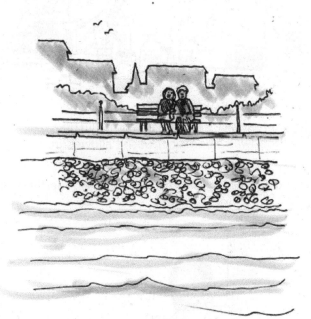

Roopwati takes an active role and has been instrumental in helping make her community become more dementia-accessible. Cuthy empowers and supports Roopwati whilst living with an ongoing physical condition.

'Oi! What are you doing in here?'

'OK, OK, I'm going.'

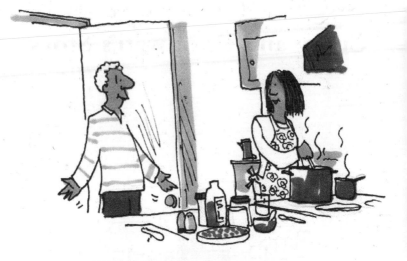

Although I was a chef, at home the kitchen was Roopwati's domain. I wasn't allowed in.

With her Guyanese influences, she was a wonderful cook.

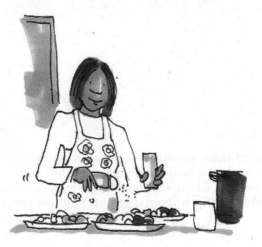

'Looks and smells fab, Roopwati!'

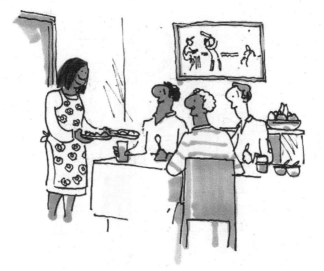

In particular, my cricket teammates enjoyed many of her feasts.

Then things changed, and I became the main cook with my Jamaican influences.

'Could you peel the potatoes?'

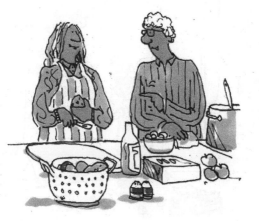

'Carrots next?'

'OK.'

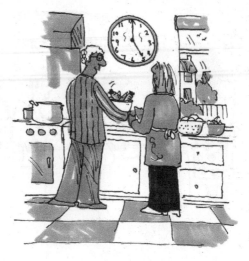

Sometimes, carrying out everyday tasks in sequence became difficult for her, but it was important that she was involved.

Tests and scans had shown she had vascular dementia.

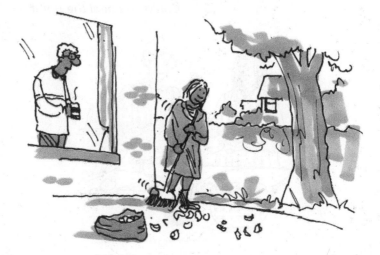

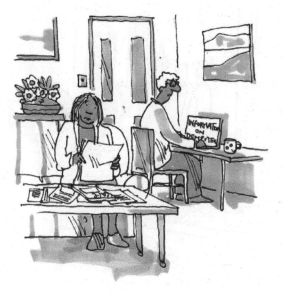

There was so much information; we were overwhelmed.

I was offered a course for dementia carers. I learnt such a lot about planning ahead, day-to-day living and entitlements.

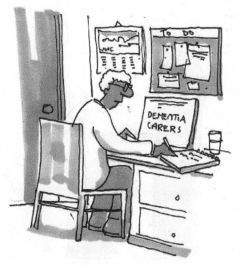

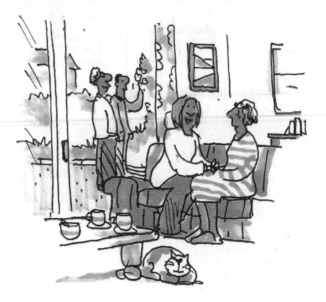

In a way, we were aware of what would happen. We had two friends who had lived with dementia and who we visited often.

Roopwati was offered medication and, although the dementia won't go away, it does help with some of the symptoms.

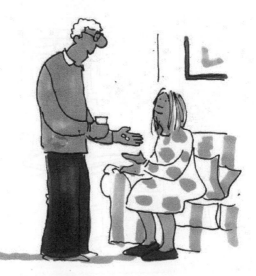

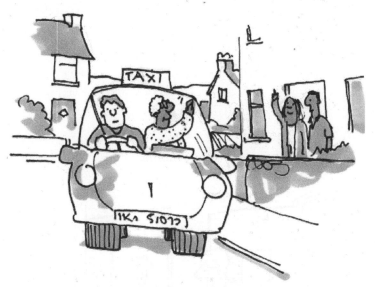

It doesn't help that I have kidney failure.

I have dialysis three times a week. It's routine for me.

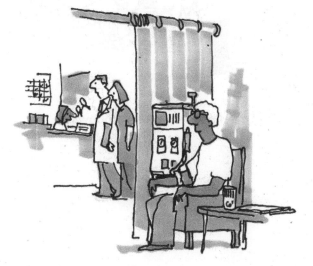

'Hi, I'm home.'

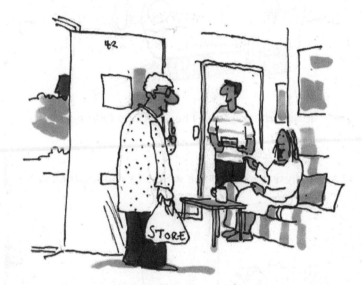

Then I get back to my Roopwati.

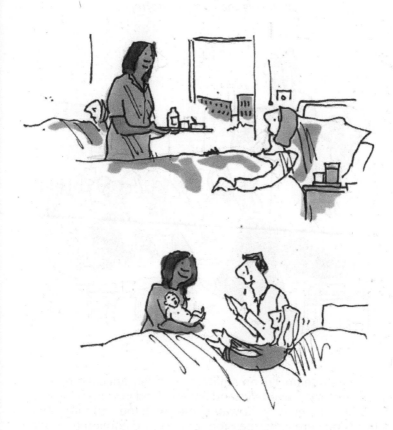

She was a nurse and a midwife, always looking after others.

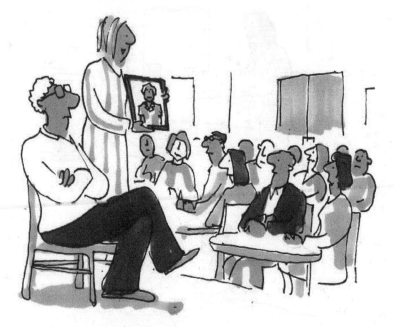

We're a team. I'm an amateur historian, specialising in black history. I give talks and am involved in various projects raising awareness. Roopwati comes with me and talks about her nursing career, her passion for care and coming to England when she was eighteen. You see, her long-term memory is good.

'Where are the toilets? How can I get help?'

Roopwati was invited to take an active part in helping our community become dementia-accessible.

Clear signage is vitally important.

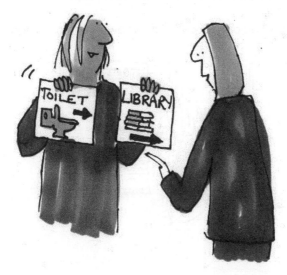

'What's that?'

'It's a mat, Roopwati.'

'Oh, I thought it was water.'

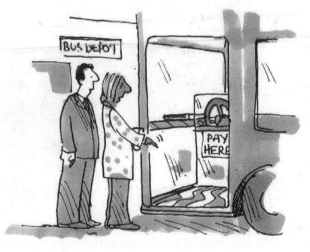

She helped with public transport, too. It can be very confusing and scary getting from A to B if you have dementia.

Roopwati isn't afraid of giving her opinion either.

'This is so confusing. I don't know where to start . . . '

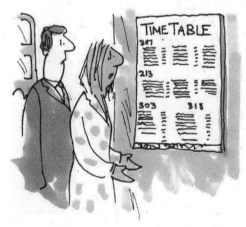

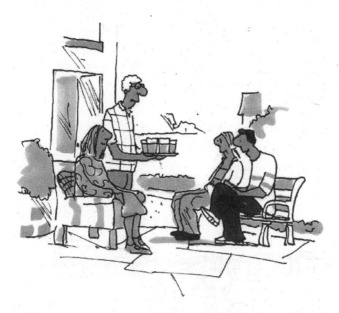

We don't want to bother anyone, and of course our children help when they can.

We enjoy our time together, but we know that when we'll need it, there is help out there.

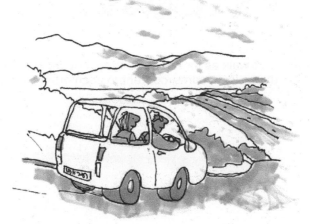

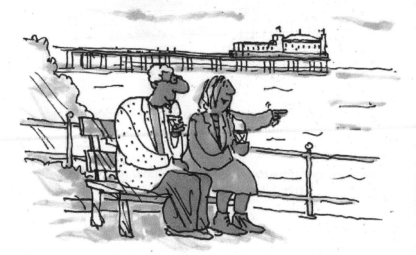

Roopwati can't walk as far as she used to, but we love to sit by the pier with our ice creams, content in each other's company.

Sienna's Story

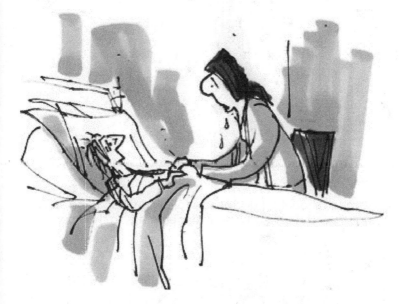

Sienna had worked in care homes in the past but, after her Gran who lived with dementia died, she wanted to give back to the community and make a meaningful difference.

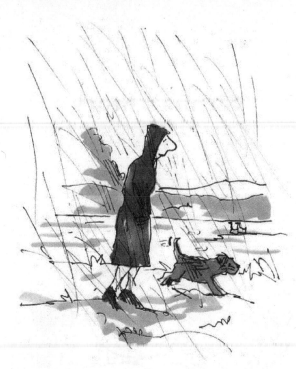

After much thought, I decided to follow my heart and started working with families living with dementia, in their homes.

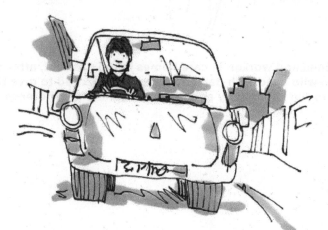

'He's been waiting for you.'

'Hi Roy, good to see you.'

'Hi.'

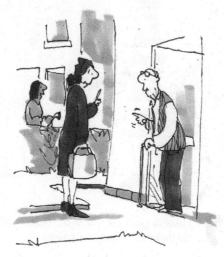

Roy is a kind, gentle man, living on his own with no family.
He has vascular dementia.

He looks forward to my visits.

'Ha ha, when I see you, it always reminds me to feed the fish.'

'That's good. I'll make a cuppa.'

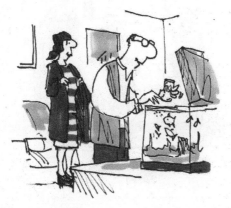

'Shall we sit in the garden, Roy? It's a gorgeous day.'

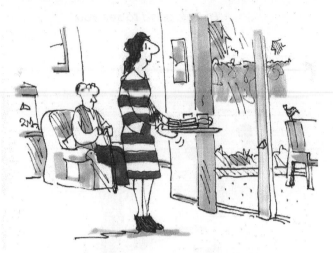

A good chat is always part of my visit, especially when I bring his favourite cake.

'Listening to the birds makes me happy.'

'Me too.'

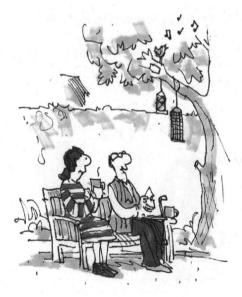

'He'll be fine, don't worry. I always check to see how he is.'

'Thanks so much.'

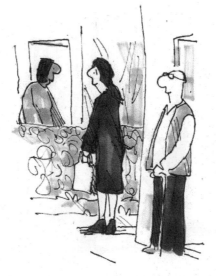

His lovely neighbour watches out for him.

The next stop is at Julia and Tim's, where I am greeted by their children, Bob and Jas. Julia has young onset dementia and was diagnosed at forty-two.

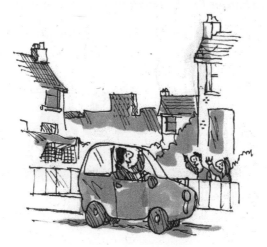

'That colour suits you, Mummy.'

'Yes, darling, it's my favourite.'

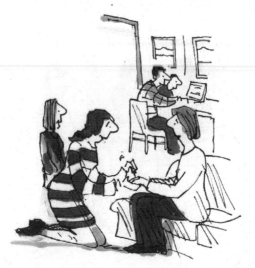

Julia is now in her mid-forties. Tim cares for her with the children.

Tim and I always have a catch-up so I can check to see how they are all coping. He works from home, which can be difficult. Fortunately, his employer is very understanding.

'It's getting harder for the children, but they're doing their best.'

'Would you like me to have a talk with them?'

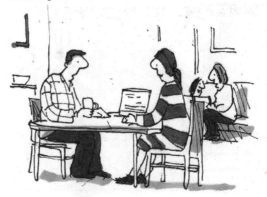

'Bob and Jas, can I have a chat about your mum's dementia?'

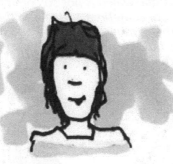

'Molly at school says Mummy will forget my name.'

'She couldn't find the bathroom yesterday. I had to take her to it.'

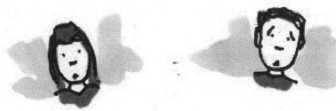

'. . . and Billy Hill said she's pretending as only old people get dementia.'

'She says the same things again and again.'

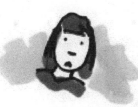

'Dementia affects the way people think, talk and act. Anyone can get dementia, not just older people. Your mummy has young onset dementia, which is not so common. Maybe I can come into the school sometime and talk to the children and teachers to help them understand more about it? Mummy may forget your name, but she won't forget how you made her feel. She loves you both very much.'

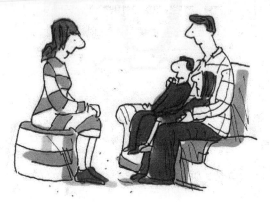

'What happens with people living with dementia is that they forget what they said, which is why Mummy says the same thing lots of times. Her brain doesn't realise that she's said it. This is why Mummy forgot where the bathroom was yesterday. She needs you – her little helpers. Maybe one of you could draw a picture of a toilet and stick it on the door? This will help her remember where it is.'

'Ah, there it is.'

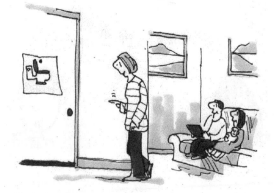

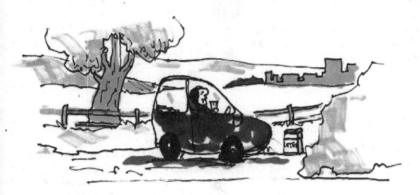

I always make sure I take a break during the day.

'Hi.'

'Hi, Sienna.'

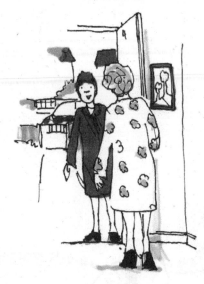

My final call is at Miriam and Jacob's. Jacob has Alzheimer's and multiple sclerosis and is nearing the end of his life.

Jacob wishes to die at home. Miriam wants to honour his wishes and I'm here to help them through.

'OK, I'll nip to the shops and meet my sisters for a coffee.'

'Great, we'll be fine. See you later.'

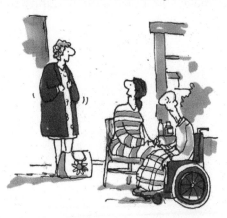

'You are a child of the universe, no less than the trees and the stars; you have a right to be here . . . '

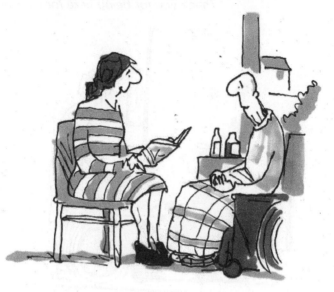

He loves me reading poetry, with 'Desiderata' a favourite.

He also loves rock 'n' roll and comes alive when I play music for him.

'Woohoo!!'

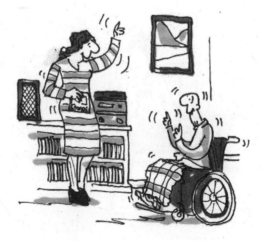

'See you in a couple of days, Jacob.'

'Thank you for being here for us, Sienna.'

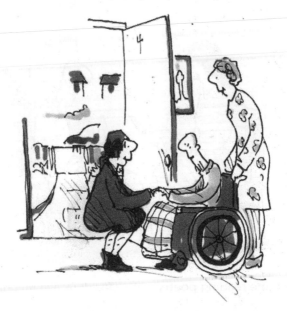

My gran always used to say to me that 'giving makes me smile inside'. I know exactly what she meant, as I feel a warm glow from within. I've found my purpose.

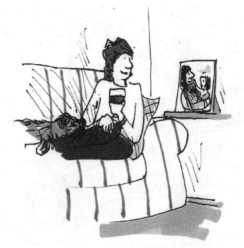

Kay, Ashley and Thomas's Story

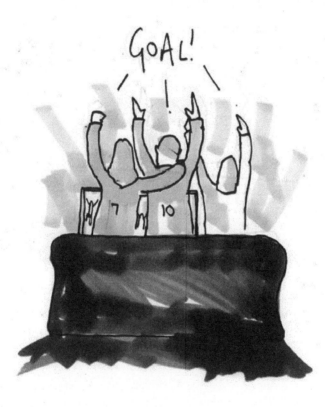

Thomas was diagnosed with young onset dementia at fifty-eight.

Thomas and Kay worked full time. Thomas was uncomfortable with carers coming in, so Kay took a different route.

'Are you OK? Is anything wrong?'

'No, nothing, nothing . . . leave me, will you?!'

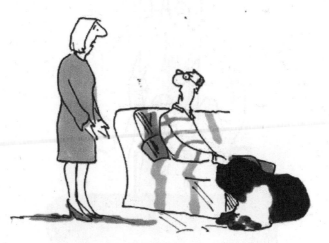

Thomas was changing. He was moody and grumpy. It was not like him at all.

*'This rota you did doesn't make any sense.
It's confusing for everyone.'*

'Well, you do it if you can do any better!'

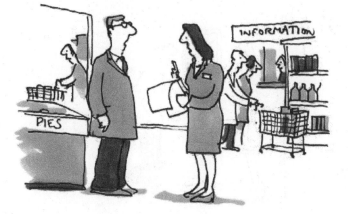

He was finding it difficult at work too.

They had no patience with him. It was so bad that, on one occasion, a customer complained about the loud dressing down Thomas was given.

'How many times do you need telling? Are you stupid?'

'Sorry, really sorry!'

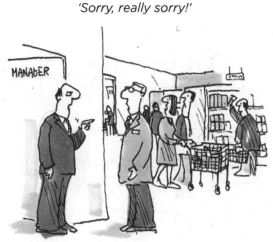

'What are you doing?'

'I'm going out, I told you.'

'No you didn't, you're lying!'

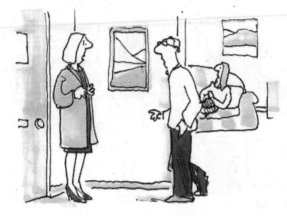

He hated me going out anywhere.

Just seeing friends became so stressful.

'Don't worry, I won't be long, I promise.'

'I don't want you to go . . . please!'

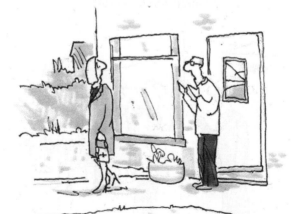

'Good night . . . '

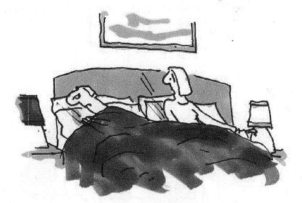

There was no intimacy any more.

Sometimes, he'd wake in a panic, not knowing where he was.

'Where am I? Where is this?!'

'You're at home. It's OK, you're safe.'

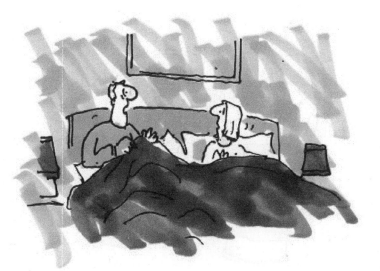

'Are you OK, Mum?'

'No, I'm not. I don't know what to do. Something's wrong.
It's like your dad doesn't want to be with me.'

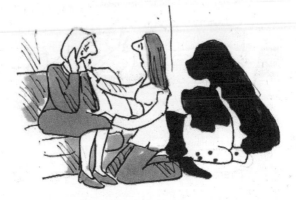

I was struggling, feeling emotionally drained and exhausted.
Our daughter Ashley had noticed.

Thomas began having tests, but nothing showed
up on the scans.

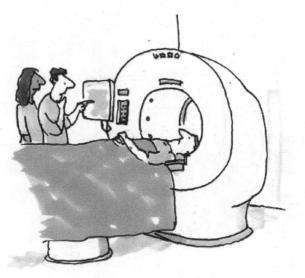

'Can we go, please? I don't want to be here. Why are we here?'

'It's OK. It will be OK.'

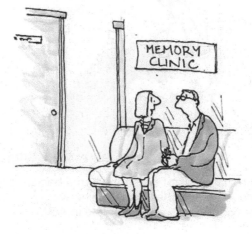

We went to the memory clinic, but he was so anxious and wanted to leave.

It was obvious Thomas was really struggling with his memory. One test was to draw a circle. He couldn't.

'I'm not sure. This is hard . . . '

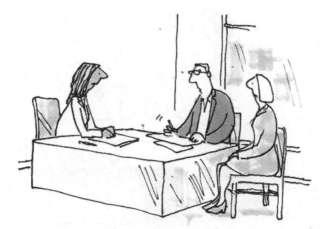

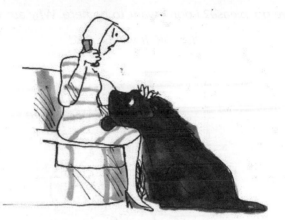

When the diagnosis of dementia came back, I rang our children Alice and then Ashley, who was on holiday, staying with her brother Tee in Australia.

At first I was working full time, so I had to get carers in, which he initially accepted in our home but, as he deteriorated, he became unsettled with them.

'Right, Thomas, time for a nice relaxing bath.'

'Go away! I don't want a bath!'

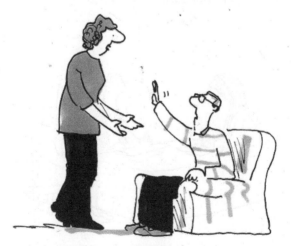

'He just won't respond to me.
He just wants his family around him, I'm sorry.'

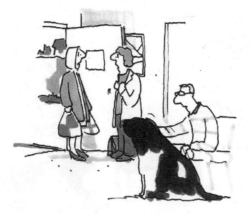

It was not working with the carers. They were nice,
but Thomas seemed anxious.

I pleaded with the council to let me become his full-time carer,
but they wouldn't budge.

'Surely it makes sense? I'm the only one he trusts.'

'No, I'm sorry, we can't sanction that.'

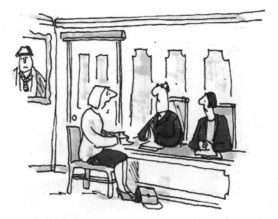

'OK, dinner's up. C'mon, move, dog!'

'Goodie, I'm hungry.'

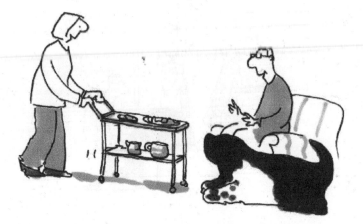

Eventually, though, the council conceded. I became Thomas's full-time carer and he was so much happier.

So, with Ashley, we began to look at making him feel as comfortable and safe as possible. And so, 'Wingit Care Home' was born!

'Come on, United!'

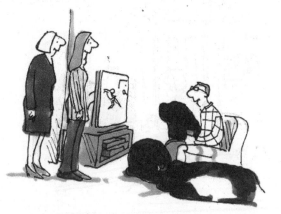

Ashley decided to forgo her career after university and help her mum and dad at home.

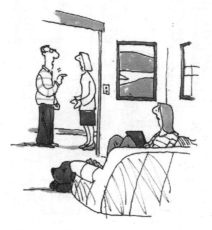

I had noticed a change in Dad. He became restless, forgetful and very isolated. When Mum tried to sort this out, it invariably ended up in a row.

Things seemed strained between them. They had been so close . . . I was scared they would split up.

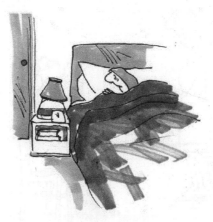

'Mum, go to bed – you look shattered!'

'Thank you, yes, I am.'

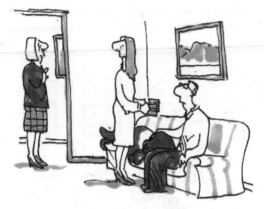

He seemed to be getting worse. Mum worked nights
and she was exhausted. When I left college,
I took a part-time job so I could help out.

My dad would often tell me how important Mum was, even
when I was taking care of him.

'You know I couldn't survive without your mum, don't you?'

'Oh really, Dad . . . here's your dinner.'

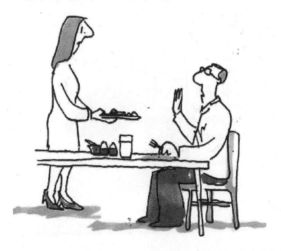

'C'mon, Ashley!'

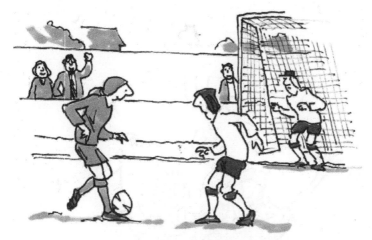

I played football to a high standard.
Mum and Dad came to all the games to support me.

But as Dad deteriorated, he stopped coming to the matches.
I missed him, but Mum was always there.

'Great goal!'

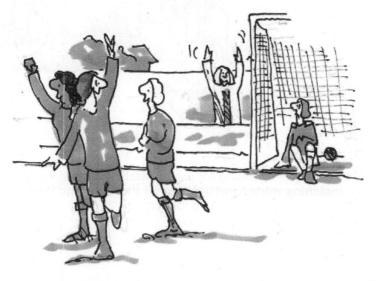

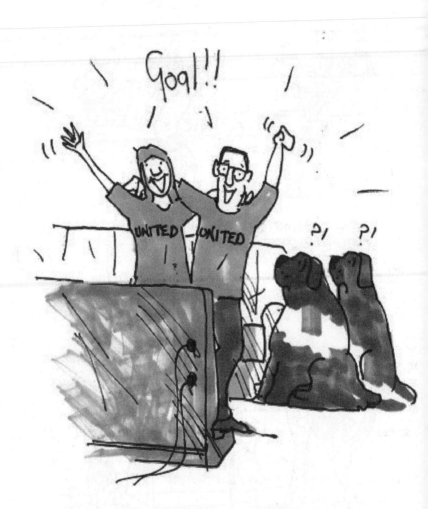

Football was bonding for us . . . watching United in our matching shirts together, sharing the highs and lows of being a football fan.

'Hi!'

'Hello!'

'Hiya!'

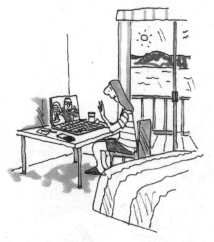

I went on a trip to Australia. Mum wanted me to have a life – she was worried about me. I kept in touch up to four times a day on FaceTime. I was frightened that Dad would forget who I was.

I was still in Australia when Mum rang to tell me Dad had been diagnosed with dementia. I wasn't surprised, but at least it was confirmed now.

'Oh, Mum . . . send Dad all my love and a big hug.'

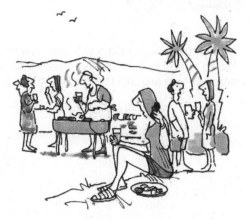

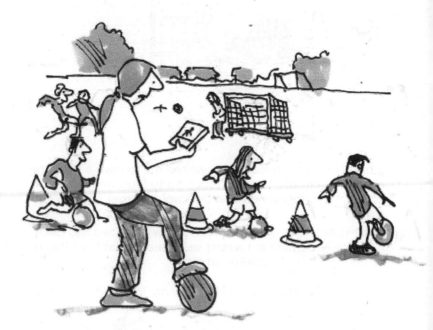

When I came back from Australia, I worked as a football coach,
but I was able to keep track of Dad's movements because we
had cameras set up around the house. It was so useful.

'They said OK!'

'Yes!'

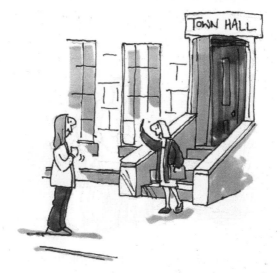

When Mum finally convinced the authorities, after a number of attempts, to make her a full-time paid carer, life became better and easier.

After such a long time, I felt that I could go out and socialise with my friends without too much worry.

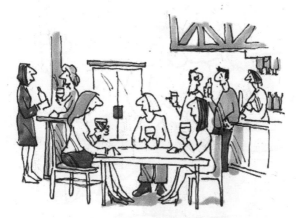

'Dad, this is Matt. He's a golfer.'

'Really, lad? Well come in, let's chat!'

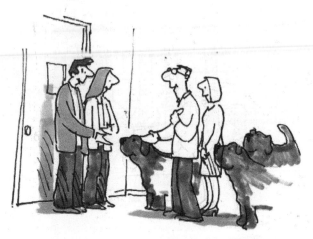

I found a lovely boyfriend, who Dad took to immediately.

Matt is brilliant with Dad – so empathetic. He understood that Dad could repeat the same questions again and again.

'Do you play golf at all?'

'Yes I do, I love it.'

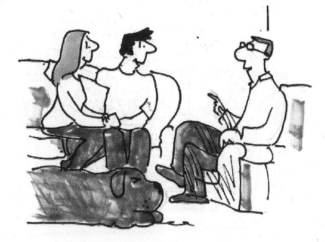

'You know I won't be able to walk my girls down the aisle, or ever hold my grandchildren . . . '

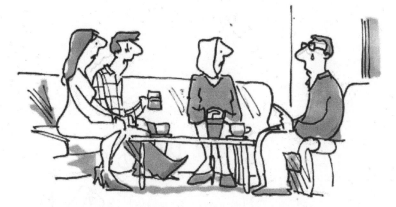

One night, Matt, my sister and I were with Dad. Mum was out. He seemed deeply thoughtful, and his lips trembled before he spoke. His eyes filled with tears . . .

It was devastating to hear, and we were still all sobbing when Mum returned. It struck home.

'Oh my, what's happened?'

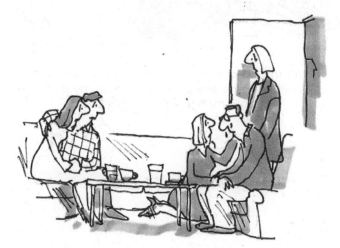

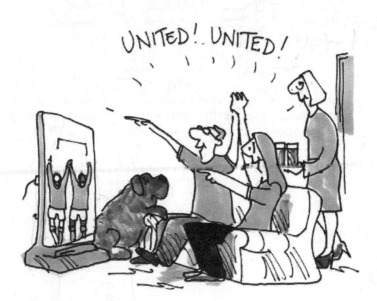

Throughout my twenties, I'd been helping to care for Dad, but I wouldn't have had it any other way. I love my dad . . . that's what matters. We are UNITED!

Part 3 of 3 – Kay, Ashley and Thomas

Thomas, Kay, Ashley and the family were 'united' as a team.

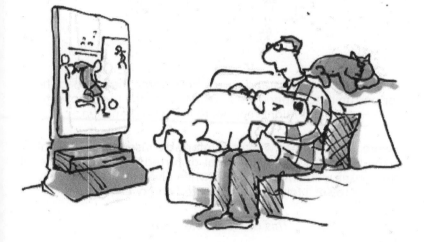

We wanted to make Thomas feel as comfortable as possible - surrounded by the familiar and, of course, love and care.

'Here, Kay, you'll need to wear these gloves.'

'Thank you.'

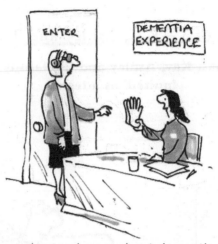

I needed to understand more about dementia and had the opportunity to experience a virtual dementia tour, replicating what it might feel like to live with dementia.

I wore gloves, shoes with uncomfortable inserts, ear defenders to muffle sound, and glasses that distorted my view. This meant my senses were impacted, and when given instructions to fold a towel, I felt confused, scared and overwhelmed.

'This is impossible! Sigh . . .'

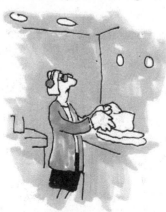

'Hi, I'm back.'

'Hello! Did you have a nice time?'

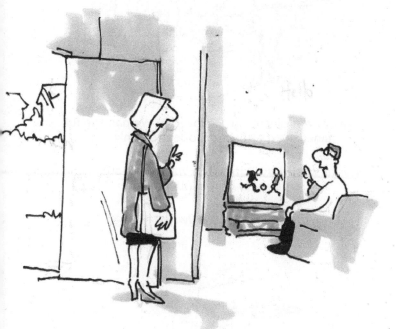

It helped me understand what it must be like for Thomas – how he saw, what he heard – and it made a huge difference to me knowing how he might feel. I recommend it to everyone.

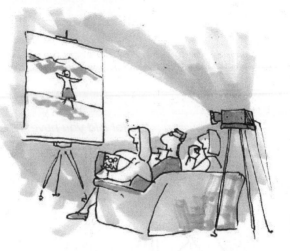

We got a projector in. He loved it. We had the full
cinema experience – popcorn, drinks . . .

His favourite was *Harry Potter*. We watched it again and again.
The fantasy of it captivated him.

'Look! He's flying!'

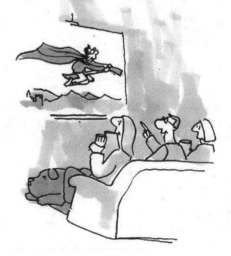

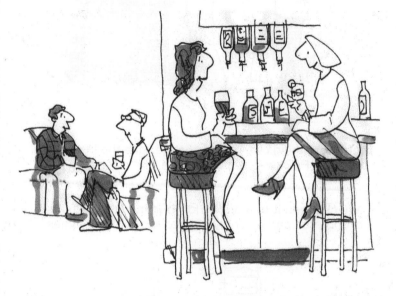

Thomas still worried when I went out. He felt vulnerable knowing I wasn't at home. So we created a bar setting in the conservatory, which meant I could invite friends. It was especially lovely when Alice and James came down from the Lake District to relax and chat.

'Don't go near there! You could fall in!'

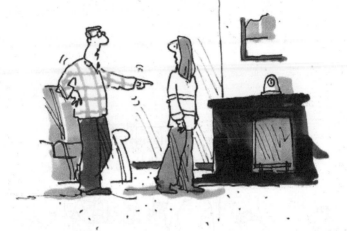

There were things we had to change. Like the black slate fireplace. He saw it as a black hole, and it terrified him.

We changed it to a bright, log-burning fire. His fears evaporated and he enjoyed watching the real flames.

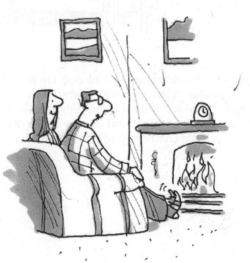

'Thomas, time for your sandwiches in the fridge.'

'Thank you, Alexa.'

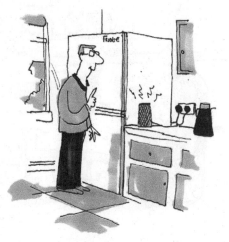

Alexa came in handy. We programmed her to prompt and remind Thomas if we were out.

But sadly, as his dementia progressed, he didn't understand Alexa's instructions.

'Thomas, time for your juice in the fridge. Thomas, time for . . . '

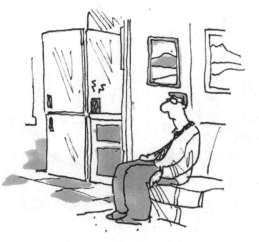

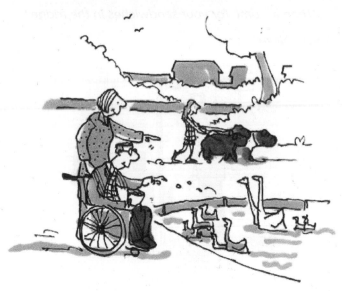

Going for strolls in the country or to the park was enjoyable and refreshing, though Thomas needed a wheelchair for longer walks.

Our pets became so important. He'd never been one for pets, but as his dementia advanced, he reached out to them. Their unconditional love touched him.

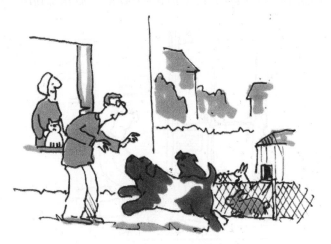

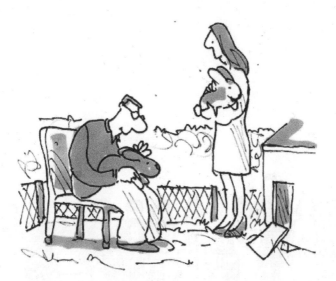

They helped calm and settle him . . . it was lovely to see.

As a family, we're all in this together, caring for Thomas with the love he deserves.

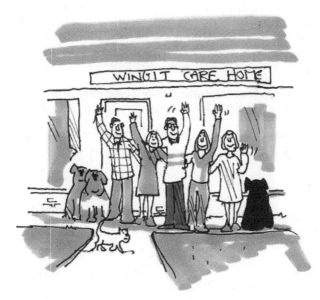

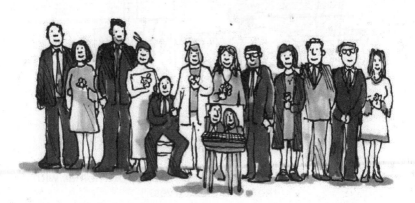

In the past, Thomas had asked me to marry him, but I said we were happy as we were. Then recently, he asked again . . . it seemed like the right time.

We had the perfect intimate family ceremony at home with Tee, our son, as Thomas's best man on Zoom from Australia.

That day, I fell in love with Thomas all over again.

Reflections

I hope the stories of my loving contributors have made a difference. The themes woven through their stories have a timeless appeal, and are based on their closest relationships. I was able to reach beneath the surface and see the complex issues faced by families – the losses, the rewards, the guilt, the love and the companionship. And while I did hear about the practical challenges faced, such as the difficulty of navigating the benefit system, I was also inspired by the humour shown against the odds and the joy found in nature, pets, music and children.

And what have I learned?

I learned about the dangers of repeatedly heading a football and how it can result in the neurodegenerative disease chronic traumatic encephalopathy (CTE), which can lead to dementia. Research continues into this.

I learned how young onset dementia can impact on a family and how critical communication is with children. Dementia does not just affect older people as I once thought. Around 3.9 million people under the age of sixty-five live with dementia worldwide.

I learned that planning ahead, including end-of-life planning, is important for all of us so we can get on with the business of living.

Dementia-accessible communities are a personal passion. For a community to be dementia-friendly, people living with dementia and their loved ones should always be at the start and heart of change. I am under no illusions about how complex dementia can be, but strongly believe that understanding comes out of sharing the lived experience. That is what we have attempted to do with this book.

The greatest thing I have learnt over the years is the emotional connection we create when we can simply 'be in the moment' with our loved ones. I have felt this, witnessed this, and to me this is the essence of connecting in a meaningful way that goes beyond words.

I would like to salute everyone in the dementia world who I have met in the past decade. You continue to teach me daily what it means to live with dementia. You enable my ongoing learning. And you constantly inspire me to continue waving the flag and working to make a difference.

Recently, working with a group of third-year medical students, I invited Dory to share some of her lived experience with young onset dementia, diagnosed at fifty-nine years old, nine years earlier. As we closed, she offered the following quote:

'We are all unique and beautiful, but together we are a masterpiece.'

Thank you, Dory, for all you do.

I truly hope this book inspires you to learn more about dementia, what caring for and supporting our loved ones means, and how unique – yet similar – each personal experience is. Let's reflect on how we can collectively and individually play our part, remembering it is the small things that make the biggest difference.

For Thomas and his beautiful family. Thomas died peacefully at home as we were nearing the end of writing this book. Thank you so much, Kay, for sharing your story and allowing me to change the end to reflect your marriage just a few weeks before.

Acknowledgements

I would like to thank the wonderful contributors and those who helped me find them – Pippa Kelly, Sarah Merriman, Rachel Yates-Hoyles, Rachel Niblock, Fran Hamilton and Ripaljeet Kaur.

Sir Malcolm Walker for the foreword and for making such an enormous difference for dementia research.

My fabulous friend Debbie Jacka for taking time out to proofread when I gave her very little notice.

Jo Earlam, you continue to make a remarkable difference for dementia through your personal experience and tremendous courage. Our illuminating conversations, sat in your conservatory and putting the world to rights, always fill me with inspiration and I often find myself wanting to skip to my car.

Colin Bray for being there on my journey. I consider you to be both an exceptional mentor and friend.

Editor Andrew McAleer, for your patience and understanding with my never-ending questions of curiosity, always handled with impeccable diplomacy – not to be underestimated.

My mum, dad, son and sister for your practical support, encouragement and love.

My dear circle of friends who embrace my eccentric, quirky ways; you keep me grounded and know who you are.

My gorgeous cockapoo River, who spent many hours laying beside me or at my feet as I tapped into my creativity, ensuring intermittently he got his regular walks and dips in the River Exe. You're the best companion I could ask for.

The people and families affected by dementia, who I learn from daily.

All of you who read and gain from my book.

And finally, Tony Husband for bringing my book alive with such incredible illustrations. You offer the most unique talent that cannot be matched. I'm so glad we met when we did.

'It's not enough to stare up the steps – we must step up the stairs'
Dr Vance Havner

Thank you all from the bottom of my heart as I continue to step up the stairs.

Resources

Below is a list of useful resources, but it is by no means exhaustive.

Alzheimer's Society
Dementia affects people differently. Find out how the Alzheimer's Society can support you by phone, online or face-to-face.
www.alzheimers.org.uk

Alzheimer's Research UK
Finding a cure for the diseases that cause dementia.
www.alzheimersresearchuk.org

Beth Britton
Former carer to her dad, blogger, trainer, speaker and campaigner.
www.d4dementia.com

BRACE Alzheimer's Research
An independent charity committed to defeating dementia through scientific research.
www.alzheimers-brace.org

Carers UK
For help and advice – making life better for carers.
www.carersuk.org

Dementia Carers Count
Working for a world where all family and friends taking care of someone with dementia feel confident, supported and heard.
www.dementiacarers.org.uk

Dementia UK

Helping families face dementia, including young onset dementia, and providing specialist Admiral Nurses.

www.dementiauk.org

Devon Carers

Providing unpaid carers in Devon with the information and advice they need in their caring role.

www.devoncarers.org.uk

Dr Jane Mullins, dementia nurse specialist

Author of *Finding the Light in Dementia*, a guide for families, friends and caregivers.

www.findingthelightindementia.com

Dr Kathryn Mannix

Retired palliative care doctor – author of *With the End in Mind* and *Listen*.

www.withtheendinmind.co.uk

Empowered Conversations

Offering one-to-one support, communication training courses and engagement sessions for families, friends and professionals.

www.empowered-conversations.co.uk

Health Education England (HEE)

HEE exists for one reason only: to support the delivery of excellent healthcare.

www.hee.nhs.uk

Hilary Cragg

Solicitor and author of *Compassion with Dementia*.

www.hilarycragg.com/book

Innovations in Dementia

Supporting people with dementia to live with hope and keep control of their lives.

www.innovationsindementia.org.uk

John's Campaign

A campaign for the right to stay with people with dementia in hospital and care homes, and for people with dementia to be supported by their family carers.

www.johnscampaign.org.uk

Living with Dementia Toolkit

This co-produced resource is based on research evidence from the IDEAL project and the lived experience of people with dementia and carers.

www.livingwithdementiatoolkit.org.uk

Memory Matters South West

Therapeutic approaches to memory loss and dementia.

www.memorymatters.org.uk

Mycarematters

Practical solutions making a tangible difference to the quality of life of caring staff and those they care for.

www.mycarematters.org

My Future Care Handbook and Buddy Service

Support to think about and make plans for the future.

www.myfuturecare.org

NHS UK

Learn more about Chronic Traumatic Encephalopathy (CTE).

www.nhs.uk/conditions/chronic-traumatic-encephalopathy

Pippa Kelly

Dementia campaigner, journalist and podcaster raising awareness of dementia.

www.pippakelly.co.uk

Skills for Care
Helping create a well-led, skilled and valued adult social care workforce.
www.skillsforcare.org.uk

Social Care Institute for Excellence
Training, guidance and information for care staff, friends and family.
www.scie.org.uk

3SpiritUK
Training and visual learning resources about dementia.
www.3SpiritUK.com

The Filo Project
Supports individuals across Devon and Somerset, many of whom are experiencing symptoms associated with moderate dementia.
www.thefiloproject.co.uk

The Royal College of Nursing
Professional resources for dementia.
www.rcn.org.uk/clinical-topics/dementia/professional-resources

Together In Dementia Everyday (Tide)
Tide is a UK-wide network connecting carers and former carers of people with dementia to create lasting change together.
www.tide.uk.net

Training 2 Care
Virtual Dementia Tour.
www.training2care.com/virtual-dementia-tour.htm

Wendy Mitchell
Blogger on living day to day with dementia. Bestselling author of *Somebody I Used To Know* and *What I Wish People Knew About Dementia*.
whichmeamitoday.wordpress.com

Gina Awad

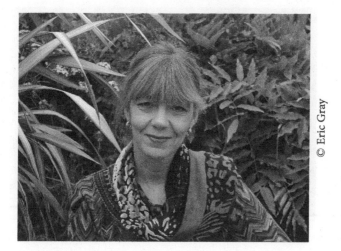

© Eric Gray

Gina Awad has been involved in working to make a difference for people living with dementia and their loved ones for over a decade. As well as becoming the Alzheimer's Society's Dementia Friends Champion of the Year in 2016 and forming the Exeter Dementia Action Alliance, she was also awarded a British Empire Medal for her voluntary services to people with dementia and their families in Devon in 2018. Gina has a BSc in Health & Social Care from the Open University, is a qualified counsellor, reflexologist and coach, and gained great insight when she was awarded a scholarship to the Memory Bridge Training Retreat at the Tibetan Mongolian Buddhist Cultural Center in Bloomington, Indiana. She believes that end-of-life planning is essential in enabling people to consider their future decisions before getting back to the joys and challenges of daily living. Gina has personal experience of family and friends living with dementia and hosts the 'Living Better with Dementia' radio show on Exeter-based radio station Phonic 106.8 FM.

Tony Husband

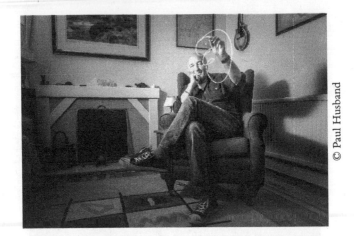

© Paul Husband

Tony Husband is a multi-award-winning cartoonist. He draws for *Private Eye* and many other publications. His book *Take Care, Son* about his father's journey through dementia has led him into the dementia world, and he's worked on dementia-awareness projects all over the UK. His dementia poems have been turned into songs, and he has just finished a short film, *Joe's Journey*, starring Sir Tony Robinson and based on his story of a man living with dementia.